Antioxidants

Natural Defense
Against Oxidative Stress

GW00776534

Barbara Wexler, MPH

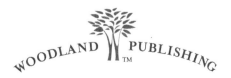

WOODLAND PUBLISHING TM

For ordering information and bulk order discounts, contact:
Woodland Publishing, 448 East 800 North, Orem, UT 84097
Toll-free telephone: (800) 777-BOOK

Please visit our Web site: www.woodlandpublishing.com

Note: The information in this book is for educational purposes only and is not recommended as a means of diagnosing or treating an illness. All matters concerning physical and mental health should be supervised by a health practitioner knowledgeable in treating that particular condition. Neither the publisher nor the author directly or indirectly dispenses medical advice, nor do they prescribe any remedies or assume any responsibility for those who choose to treat themselves.

A cataloging-in-publication record for this book is available from the Library of Congress.

ISBN: 978-1-58054-427-6

Printed in the United States of America

Contents

The Perils of Oxidative Stress

Many of the body's natural biological processes create harmful by-products including toxic chemicals called free radicals. These byproducts, collectively referred to as oxidants, can set up chain reactions in the body that damage cells, block the action of critical enzymes and interfere with a wide variety of healthy cellular processes. Oxidants can injure our cell membranes, damage DNA—our core genetic material—interfere with the proper division and replication of cells and block the generation of energy the body needs to run.

In addition to oxidants that arise from natural biological processes, many other factors including stress, illness and poor nutrition can create additional oxidants. Free radicals also are produced in response to environmental exposures such as cigarette smoke, air pollution, insecticides, some fried or burnt foods, alcohol, radiation, chemicals and environmental toxins.

Taken together, these factors can create a condition in the body referred to as "oxidative stress." While oxidative stress is not itself a disease, high levels of unresolved oxidative stress can weaken the body and contribute to the development of many serious illnesses, especially those of a chronic or degenerative nature.

For example, free radicals can increase the harmful actions of low-density lipoprotein (LDL is the "bad" cholesterol linked to increased risk for heart disease). Because free radicals are also believed to be instrumental in the development of chronic diseases such as cancer, heart disease, cataracts, and may even accelerate aging, antioxidants may play an important role in disease prevention.

With advancing age, the body's tissues and cells become more susceptible to free radical attacks and damage from oxidative stress. Oxidative stress has been implicated as a factor contributing to the development of more than thirty different disorders—from heart disease and stroke to Alzheimer's disease and cancer.

The Importance of Antioxidants

Fortunately, the body is poised to effectively respond to the damage caused by free radicals and other oxidizing chemicals. Antioxidants are chemical scavengers that bind to harmful oxidants and neutralize them. In a sense, antioxidants are chemical decoys that allow themselves to become the targets of oxidation, thus sparing our vital tissues and important chemical reactions from damage. Antioxidants help our bodies deal with oxidative stress caused by free radical damage.

We've all heard that antioxidants are important to our health. But if we look closely at the word *antioxidant* it may seem like a paradox. After all, oxygen is essential to our well being. Why should we want to oppose it with an antioxidant? Breathing oxygen connects us to life. If the brain is deprived of oxygen for more than a few minutes, irreparable damage occurs, followed by death. So why should the body need an abundance of antioxidants—chemicals that fight the effects of oxygen?

The answer to this question lies in the subtle but essential distinction between oxygenation and oxidation, a truly profound difference that takes us back to the evolutionary roots of the one hundred trillion cells in our bodies. The two-faced nature of oxygen—on the one hand an essential nutrient that we can't live without, and on the other a savage destroyer that must be blocked and opposed—is known as the oxygen paradox.

The Oxygen Paradox

The human body thrives in the presence of oxygen. Our cells burn sugars and fats in the presence of oxygen through an incredibly efficient aerobic (oxygen utilizing) biochemical process called the Krebs cycle (also called the citric acid cycle or the tricyclic acid (TCA) cycle). This constructive use of oxygen to generate cellular energy is called oxygenation. As long as oxygen is carefully directed into aerobic biochemical processes like the Krebs cycle, it's truly the body's best friend.

The diagram to the right provides a glimpse into the complexity of the

Krebs cycle which, in turn, is just a small part of the network of chemical reactions that make up our human metabolism and internal biological terrain.

But oxygen has another face, one we see everyday whenever we look at metallic objects that have been left out in the elements to weather and rust. Oxygen is a highly reactive, corrosive chemical. It can turn the strongest iron chain into a weak and crumbling wreck by corrupting it, one atom at a time, through a process known as *oxidation*.

Oxidation is a process in which oxygen (or certain other chemicals) attach themselves to other substances by stripping away their electrons. In the case of rust, oxygen attaches to iron to form oxide compounds that weaken and corrode the original structure.

Inside the living body, something very similar can take place. Oxygen is capable of stripping an electron from another biochemical—effectively changing it into a positively charged ion since it has given up a negatively charged electron.

Sometimes this positive ion attaches to the oxygen or another negatively charged material. But on other occasions, the positively charged ion—which is now hungry for an electron so it can get back into electrical balance—strips an electron from a neighboring molecule, balancing itself but creating a new, imbalanced ion. The newly stripped ion can repeat this process and, like a line of dominos falling over, each one knocking down the next, a long chain of chemical changes can take place, each one damaging and degrading a previously balanced and functional biochemical substance.

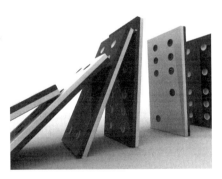

Driving Between the Lines

As long as the oxygen within our bodies is directed into aerobic processes like the Krebs cycle, everything works perfectly. It's like cars speeding down the highway at 60 miles an hour. As long as they stay in their lanes, traffic flows along nicely and everyone travels smoothly and safely.

But if the system of lanes breaks down and cars start weaving and moving around in every possible direction, then the situation immediately becomes dangerous and inefficient. It's the same way with oxygen, except that instead of painted lines to mark off lanes, our bodies have highly developed systems of antioxidants that try to keep atoms of oxygen traveling in the right direction—for example, into the Krebs cycle—and prevent them from making trouble elsewhere in the body. In other words, these antioxidant systems keep the body focused on oxygenation—the constructive use of oxygen—rather than oxidation.

Some of the body's major antioxidant systems include glutathione peroxidase, superoxide dismutase, catalase and cytochrome P450. Some of these substances and the biochemical pathways they define are meant to keep oxygen heading in the right direction while others aim to keep it from heading off in the wrong direction.

Here's an analogy that might help put the two faces of oxygen—the positive face of oxygenation that feeds our cells and the negative face of oxidation that stresses them—into context.

A Tale of Life Beneath the Sea

The navy has a fleet of nuclear submarines. These remarkable ships are capable of remaining submerged in the ocean for months at a time as they travel around the world. The energy needed to power these huge machines comes from compact nuclear reactors that tap the energy of atomic nuclei to generate heat. In addition to driving the sub, this heat is used for everything on board—from scrubbing and recharging the air that the seamen breathe and purifying the water they drink to running the radar and information systems that keep them in touch with the world and on track. If the nuclear generator on board were to fail, the lives of the crew would be imperiled.

On the other hand, the nuclear fuel needs to stay deep within the core of the reactor. Even though it produces the life-giving energy that every person on board depends on, the fuel itself is toxic. A few moments of direct exposure would create a lethal dose of radiation poisoning. The nuclear fuel must be kept within very specific "lanes"—in this case, the physical shielding of the reactor's core.

It's just the same with oxygen. It gives us life, but only when it is directed to and kept within the "core" of the biochemical processes that use oxygen to make energy. Just like nuclear fuel escaping from the core, oxygen that escapes from the bounds of our antioxidant systems becomes very, very dangerous to our health.

The Many Faces of Oxidative Stress

When oxygen slips outside of the lanes created in the body by antioxidants, it strips electrons from nearby substances, creating positively charged ions called free radicals. As we've described, one free radical, in an effort to find an electron to rebalance itself, damages another molecule, converting it into a free radical and so forth. This domino-like series of damaging events is known as an "oxidative stress cascade."

Oxidative damage causes many problems:

First off, through the cascade process we've just described it can break down essential substances in the body, degrading them and even turning them into toxins and wastes that must be removed from the body, rather than helpful substances that serve it.

Secondly, by locking up electrons, oxidatively damaged free radicals reduce the flow of electrons the body uses to create and direct energy at a cellular level. In traditional Chinese medicine, the term *ch'i* is used to refer to vital energy. In biochemical terms, ch'i may be understood in terms of this flow. When the body enters a highly oxidized state, electron flow, and therefore vital energy, is reduced. We may experience this as a loss of physical energy, depression, anxiety or other nervous system problems, poor digestion and a wide range of metabolic complaints ranging from constipation to diabetes. It also may manifest as weakened immunity, leading to an increased susceptibility to infections or slower recovery and healing.

Finally, the presence of free radicals in the body is a trigger for many inflammatory processes. Free radicals trigger the production of NF-κB (nuclear transcription factor kappa-B), which in turn signals the production of inflammatory cytokines—immune system substances produced by the body to fight cancer and other infections. While this can be helpful if triggered at the right time, when we are constantly exposed to oxidatively damaged free radicals, the over-expression of NF-κB and its related, downstream production of cytokines can give rise to chronic inflammatory problems including arthritic symptoms, fibromyalgia and even cardiovascular diseases.

How Our Cells Use Oxygen

With every inhalation—each breath of air we take—oxygen is drawn down into the lungs through a branching network of finer and finer tubes called bronchi. At the end of these bronchi the air inflates a spongy mass composed of billions of microscopic balloons called alveoli (singular = alveolus). Each alveolar bubble is wrapped in a network of tiny blood vessels so thin that the oxygen inside the alveoli passes directly into the blood. This oxygen-rich blood is then returned to the heart where it is pumped to all of the cells of the body.

Our cells, in turn, have the ability to absorb oxygen from the blood. One of the central biochemical processes within our cells takes this oxygen and delivers it, along with other nutrients including sugars and fats, to the energy producing centers within the cell—specialized capsules called mitochondria. Mitochondria use these nutrients as fuel to produce a molecule called adenosine triphosphate, more commonly referred to as ATP. ATP is the body's universal currency for storing and delivering energy where it's needed, for everything from running to catch a bus to processing the electrical signals in the nervous system that give rise to thought and awareness.

Free Radicals, Oxidative Stress and Disease

We know that oxidative stress is a harmful condition that can damage cells. It occurs when the balance of highly reactive, unstable molecules known as free radicals and antioxidants shifts in favor of the free radicals.

Free radicals are formed during a range of biochemical reactions and cellular functions including mito-

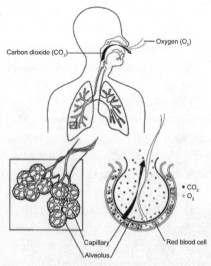

Transfer of oxygen into the blood and removal of waste carbon dixoide occurs in the alveolar tissue of the lungs

chondrial metabolism. Various conditions disrupt this balance by increasing the formation of free radicals in proportion to the available antioxidants. Oxidative stress describes the conditions, disorders and diseases that lead to and increase the formation of free radicals, inflammation, infection and cancer.

Free radicals are generally reactive oxygen or nitrogen species such as hydrogen peroxide, hydroxyl radical, nitric oxide, peroxynitrite, singlet oxygen, superoxide anion and peroxyl radical. An example of a very potent free radical is peroxynitrite, which is 1,000 times more potent as an oxidizing compound than hydrogen peroxide. Markers of peroxynitrite formation (such as nitrotyrosines or isoprostanes) have been found in many diseases including the brains of persons suffering from neurodegenerative diseases such as Alzheimer's and Parkinson's disease as well as in persons afflicted with chronic heart disease, liver disease and inflammatory conditions. Inflammation, poor blood flow, degenerative diseases and toxin exposures, among other conditions, all lead to oxidative stress. These PET scan images show the activity of a normal brain (left) versus one afflicted with Alzheimer's disease (right).

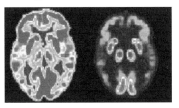

Dietary Sources of Antioxidants

So how do we get antioxidants? Fruits, vegetables and cereals, including barley, corn, millet, and oats, and legumes, including broad beans, pinto beans, and soybeans, are potent sources of antioxidant vitamins. Fruits and vegetables also contain a variety of phytonutrients that often act as antioxidants, protecting the cells of the body from the damaging effect of free radicals. Some of the best sources of antioxidants are berries, ginger, pomegranate, sunflower seeds and walnuts.

Citrus fruits and berries contain bioflavonoids such as hesperidin and anthocyanins, while vegetables such as Brussels sprouts, peppers, kale and spinach contain quercetin, apigentin, myricetin and luteolin.[1] Corn, egg yolks and green vegetables contain lutein and zeaxanthin, and meat, especially organ meat, contains alpha-lipoic acid, coenzyme Q10 and selenium.

But fruits, vegetables, cereals and legumes are not the number-one source of antioxidants in the U.S. diet because most Americans don't even come close to eating the recommended amounts of fruits and vegetables. (The 2005 Dietary

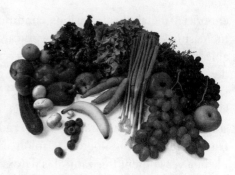

Guidelines for Americans recommend 2 to 6 1/2 cups of fruits and vegetables a day, or the equivalent of 4 to 13 servings depending on your age, gender, and activity level.)

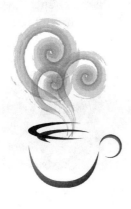

Surprisingly, coffee is the leading source of antioxidants in the U.S. diet—not because it is especially high in antioxidants, but because Americans drink so much of it. Their morning coffee gives Americans nearly 1,300 mg daily of antioxidants in the form of polyphenols. The second and third dietary sources of polyphenols in the U.S. diet are black tea (294 mg) and bananas (76 mg) followed by dry beans (72 mg/day), corn (48 mg/day), red wine (44 mg/day), beer (42 mg/day), apples (39 mg/day), tomatoes (32 mg/day), and potatoes (28 mg/day).[2]

A List of Well-Known Antioxidants

There are literally thousands of naturally occurring antioxidants. The box on page 13 lists some better-known antioxidants and the dietary sources of these nutrients.

Well-Known Antioxidants

ANTIOXIDANT	DIETARY SOURCES
Alpha-lipoic acid	Red meat, liver and yeast
Beta-carotene	Yellow, orange and green fruits and vegetables such as apricots, carrots, kale, kohlrabi, parsley, spinach and turnip greens
Coenzyme Q10	Organ meat is a potent source of CoQ10, and mackerel, peanuts, sardines, soybeans, spinach beef and chicken contain smaller amounts.
Ellagic acid	Berries, pecans, pomegranates and walnuts
Epicatechins, catechins and thearubigins	Green tea and black tea
Hesperidin	Citrus fruits are the most potent sources
Lutein and zeaxanthin	Corn, egg yolks, and green vegetables and fruits (broccoli, Brussels sprouts, kale, cabbage, green beans, green peas, spinach, kiwi, and honeydew melon)
Lycopene	Red and pink fruits including papaya, pink grapefruit, pink guava, tomatoes and watermelon
Proanthocyanins	Grape seed extract
Quercetin	Green tea, onions and red wine
Selenium	Seafood, meat, and organ meats. Plant sources such as whole grains and seeds vary in content depending on the selenium content of the soil where they were grown.
Turmeric	The spice is commonly used in curries and South Asian cuisine. Its active ingredient is curcumin.
Vitamin C	Berries, broccoli, Brussels sprouts, cabbage, citrus fruits, collard greens, cauliflower, guava, kale, melons, spinach, sweet peppers, watercress, turnip greens
Vitamin E	Unprocessed vegetable oils. Smaller amounts are found in whole grains, dark-green leafy vegetables, legumes and nuts

Types of Antioxidants

Vitamins and Cofactors

Vitamins A, B-6, B-12, C, E and folate (also knows as vitamin B9) have antioxidant properties. Vitamin A, also known as retinol, is synthesized in the body from beta-carotene, a phytonutrient that protects dark green, orange and yellow vegetables from solar radiation damage and may provide comparable protection for people. Vitamin B-6, also known as pyridoxine, is necessary for the synthesis of the neurotransmitters serotonin and norepinephrine, and for myelin formation. Sources of vitamin B-6 include carrots, cereal grains, cheese, eggs, fish, flour, legumes, liver, meat, milk, peas, potatoes and spinach.

Vitamin B-12 is an essential water-soluble vitamin found in a variety of foods such as fish, shellfish, meats, and dairy products. It helps maintain healthy nerve cells and red blood cells, and is also needed to make DNA, the genetic material in all cells.

Vitamin C, also known as ascorbic acid, is a water-soluble nutrient. Because vitamin C can donate electrons, it effectively prevents damage caused by free radicals. When you coat apple slices in lemon juice to prevent them from turning brown—oxidizing—you're seeing the antioxidant power of the vitamin C in lemon juice in action.

Vitamin E is a fat-soluble nutrient, consisting of tocopherols, especially alpha-tocopherol, that are found chiefly in plant leaves, wheat germ oil and nuts. Vitamin E is important in the formation of red blood cells and helps the body use vitamin K, and it's effective as a free radical scavenger by donating hydrogen to fatty peroxyl radicals, which halts lipid peroxidation. Experimentally, it has been shown that dietary vitamin E can prevent the development of some forms of atherosclerosis—the clogging, narrowing and hardening of blood vessels that can lead to stroke, heart attack, and eye and kidney problems.[21]

Folate and folic acid are forms of a water-soluble B vitamin. Folate occurs naturally in food, and folic acid is the synthetic form of this vitamin. Sources include asparagus, baked goods, bananas, beef liver, broccoli, cereals, legumes, lemons, lettuce, melons, mushrooms, okra, orange juice, organ meat, spinach, tomato juice and yeast. Folate helps produce and maintain new cells and also helps prevent changes to DNA that may lead to cancer.

Coenzyme Q10 (CoQ10) is a vitamin-like compound that is vital for activities related to energy metabolism. It is a potent antioxidant that is naturally present in small amounts in a variety of foods. Organ meats such as heart, liver and kidney, as well as beef, soybeans and soybean oil, sardines, mackerel, spinach and peanuts contain CoQ10. CoQ10 inhibits lipid and protein peroxidation—breaking down to form more free radicals—and scavenges free radicals. It is continually undergoing oxidation-reduction recycling. The reduced form readily gives up electrons to neutralize oxidants and displays its strongest antioxidant activity. CoQ10 is the only fat-soluble antioxidant that is synthesized in our bodies. It is also metabolized to ubiquinol, which prolongs the antioxidant effect of vitamin E.

Minerals

Manganese is an essential trace mineral that acts as a cofactor in the production of the body's most important antioxidant enzyme—superoxide dismutase. Dietary sources of manganese include whole grains, nuts, leafy vegetables and teas.

Magnesium is the fourth most abundant mineral in the body and is essential to good health. It is involved in hundreds of biochemical reactions in the body—helping to maintain normal muscle and nerve function, stabilizing heart rhythm, supporting healthy immune function and keeping bones strong. Magnesium also helps to regulate blood sugar levels, promote normal blood pressure, and is involved in energy metabolism and protein synthesis. Research suggests that magnesium may play an important role in preventing disorders such as hypertension, cardiovascular disease, and diabetes. Green vegetables such as spinach, legumes, nuts and seeds, and whole, unrefined grains are good sources of magnesium.

Selenium is an essential dietary mineral and a trace element component of several enzymes, including selenium-glutathione-peroxidase, which neutralizes hydrogen peroxide that is produced by some cell processes and if unopposed, would damage cell membranes. Selenium also is involved in stimulating antibody formation in response to vaccines and may offer protection from the toxic effects of heavy metals and other substances. The content of selenium in food depends on the selenium content of the soil where plants are grown or animals are raised.

Population studies indicate that death from cancer, including lung, colorectal, and prostate cancers, is lower among people with higher blood levels or intake of selenium. Research suggests that selenium reduces cancer risk in several ways. As an antioxidant, it can help protect the body from damaging effects of free radicals. Selenium may also prevent or slow tumor growth. Certain breakdown products of selenium are believed to prevent tumor growth by enhancing immune cell activity and suppressing development of blood vessels to the tumor.[35]

Carotenoids

Carotenoids are the natural fat-soluble pigments that provide the colors of many red, green, yellow and orange fruits and vegetables. Alpha, beta, and gamma carotene act as powerful antioxidants and are consid-

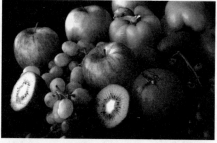

ered provitamins because they can be converted to active vitamin A. Some other well-known carotenoids are lutein, lycopene and zeaxanthin. Interestingly, the body better absorbs lycopene when it is consumed in processed tomato products rather than fresh tomatoes. The reason for this is not yet known. In one study lycopene was absorbed 2 1/2 times better from tomato paste than from fresh tomatoes. Cooking fresh tomatoes with a little oil greatly increases the bioavailability of lycopene and its absorption.

Carotenoids have been shown to reduce the risk of certain types of cancer—specifically, premenopausal breast cancer and cervical, prostate, digestive tract and lung cancers, however, their consumption by smokers has been linked to increased risk of lung cancer.[4] Other health benefits attributed to carotenoids include protection against heart disease, cataracts, and macular degeneration, improvement in blood sugar regulation and protection of nerve cells that may help to protect against Alzheimer's disease. Researchers at the University of Wisconsin in Madison found that persons aged 50 to 75 who ate a diet rich in lutein and zeaxanthin appeared to have a lower risk of intermediate age-related macular degeneration. (AMD is the leading cause of blindness among older Americans. There is no cure, and current treatments only slow the progression of the disease.) [34]

Bioflavonoids

Bioflavonoids, also known as flavonoids or catechins, are polyphenols and water-soluble pigments that appear to confer significant health benefits. More than 4,000 bioflavonoids have been identified, including anthocyanins, which give plants 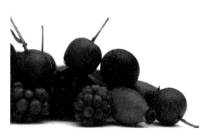 their vivid blue, purple and deep red hues and are abundant in blueberries and red grape skins.

Bioflavonoids have been termed "natural biological response modifiers" because of their ability to adapt and moderate the body's reaction to microbes—allergens, viruses, and carcinogens (cancer-causing agents). They have demonstrated anti-allergic, anti-inflammatory, antimicrobial and anticancer activity. Bioflavonoids also serve as powerful antioxidants, protecting against oxidative stress and free radical damage.

Laboratory research has demonstrated that specific bioflavonoids suppress tumor growth, prevent blood clots and have anti-inflammatory properties. Bioflavonoids are found in apples, berries, broccoli, celery, cherries, cranberries, coffee, dark chocolate, eggplant, kale, onions, parsley, pomegranate, purple grape juice, red wine, soybeans, tea, tomatoes, thyme, and walnuts.

Some of the most important bioflavonoids are resveratrol, quercetin, and catechin. There is mounting evidence that resveratrol, which is found in red wine, dark-colored grapes and olive oil, may have significant health benefits. In laboratory studies, it has been shown to increase cell survival and extend the life span of worms and fish by 60 percent and of fruit flies by 30 percent. Recent research reveals that when resveratrol was given to mice, it counteracted some of the effects of a high calorie diet and improved both their health and life span. [3]

Catechins are the primary flavonoids in tea and may be responsible for its beneficial effects. The best sources of catechins are unfermented white and green teas, which are steamed or fired to inactivate polyphenol oxidase, and then dried. As a result, white tea retains the high concentrations of catechins present in fresh tea leaves. Green tea is made from more mature tea leaves than white tea, and although it's also rich in catechins, green teas may have different catechin profiles than white teas. Bioflavonoids in dark chocolate, particularly epicatechin, may also be health protective—improving heart health and circulation.

Is Chocolate a Health Food?

Believe it or not, in terms of heart-healthy antioxidants, a dark chocolate bar packs more antioxidant punch than a bowl of blueberries or a cup of tea. Epicatechins are the bioflavonoids in chocolate that help to keep blood vessels healthy and protect against 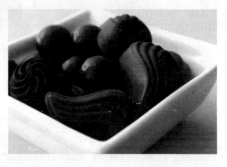 elevated LDL cholesterol, high blood pressure and unhealthy blood clotting.

In the U.S., chocolate is the third highest daily per capita dietary source of antioxidants. In an animal study of heart disease, cocoa powder at a human dose equivalent of two dark chocolate bars per day significantly inhibited atherosclerosis; lowered cholesterol, low-density lipoprotein, and triglycerides; raised high-density lipoprotein; and protected the lower-density lipoproteins from oxidation.[31]

A human study found that eating 3 1/2 ounces of dark chocolate raised blood polyphenols by nearly 20 percent, and other research reported that eating the same amount of dark chocolate every day for two weeks reduced blood pressure readings in people with high blood pressure.[18]

Another study fed different types of chocolate to healthy men and women aged 25 to 35. On some days they each ate 100 grams of dark chocolate by itself, 100 grams of dark chocolate with a small glass of whole milk, or 200 grams of milk chocolate. An hour after eating the chocolate, the subjects who ate dark chocolate alone had the most antioxidants in their blood. And they had the highest levels of epicatechins. The milk chocolate eaters had the lowest levels of epicatechins.[19]

Despite these irrefutable heart-health benefits, most nutritionists don't recommend getting all or even many of your daily antioxidants from dark chocolate because along with antioxidants, you'll get a hefty serving of sugar, saturated fat and calories. And if you gain weight, you'll offset any heart-health benefits gained by consuming antioxidants.

It's probably best to make chocolate an occasional indulgence. To satisfy your craving and reap the most health benefits, choose dark chocolate over milk chocolate. Dark chocolate contains a higher concentration of cocoa and helps to increase levels of high-density lipoproteins (HDL is the good cholesterol that confers protection against heart disease).

Isoflavones

Isoflavones, commonly known as phytoestrogens, have actions that are similar to the female hormone estrogen. Isoflavones are a subclass of bioflavonoids that includes phytoestrogens such as lignan, which is found in the fiber layers of whole grains, berries, some seeds, some vegetables and a few fruits. This class of phytonutrients may to help prevent some types of breast cancer. Flavonols such as quercetin, exert anti-inflammatory as well as antioxidant effects.[5]

Isoflavones have been shown to support healthy cholesterol, prevent bone loss, and because they keep in check enzymes that stimulate certain cancers, they act as tumor suppressors. They are predominantly concentrated in soy products, with smaller amounts found in chickpeas, flax and other seeds, barley, and milk products from cows fed on clover.

Along with its anti-inflammatory actions, quercetin also inhibits oxidation of low-density lipoprotein and appears to offer protection against cardiovascular disease. Preliminary research suggests that it exerts inhibitory effects on various types of cancer, and it may also have antiviral action. Its best-known use is in the treatment of seasonal allergies because of its antihistamine effects. Quercetin also has been found to improve the quality of life of men suffering from chronic nonbacterial prostatitis—inflammation of the prostate gland that is often painful.[6]

There also is emerging evidence that isoflavones and lignans have beneficial effects on diabetes and obesity. Research suggests that a diet rich in isoflavones and lignans improves blood glucose control and insulin resistance. In studies of people with or without diabetes, these phytonutrients appear to moderate blood sugar levels and help to reduce body weight and blood lipid levels.[7]

Isothiocyanates

Isothiocyanates and indoles are sulfur-containing phytochemicals also known as mustard oils. They give cruciferous vegetables—bok choy, broccoli, Brussels sprouts, cabbage, cauliflower, collard greens, kale, kohlrabi, rutabaga, turnips, and watercress—their sharp distinctive flavors. (Cruciferous vegetables are also high in other antioxidants such as vitamin C, and selenium.) Isothiocyanates stimulate enzymes that convert estrogen to a more benign form and may block steroid hormones that promote some breast and prostate cancers.

Isothiocyanates act by inhibiting cell proliferation associated with cancer by inducing apoptosis.[8, 9] Apoptosis is form of cell death in which a genetically programmed sequence of events leads to the elimination of cells without releasing harmful substances into the body. Apoptosis plays a key role in maintaining health by eliminating old, unnecessary and unhealthy cells.

The isothiocyanates that have demonstrated the greatest antcancer effects are phenylethylisothiocyanate, benzylisothiocyanate and 3-phenylpropylisothiocyanate. Research has revealed that isothiocyanates help to prevent lung cancer and esophageal cancer and may also reduce the risk of developing other cancers.[9]

Monoterpenes

Monoterpenes are the main components of essential oils and contain two important phytochemicals, perillyl alcohol and limonene. Limonene, found in the peel of citrus fruits, and perillyl alcohol are promising substances in cancer therapy. Present in the essential oils of citrus fruits, cherries, spearmint and dill, as well as in olive oil and canola oil, they block proteins that stimulate cell growth and reproduction and may prevent, slow or reverse the progression of some cancers as well as affect blood clotting and cholesterol. They are thought to act synergistically with other antioxidants.[10]

Organosulfurs

Organosulfurs are part of the allium family of phytochemicals. Compounds, such as allicin, may have benefits for the immune system, helping the liver to render cancer-causing substances harmless, and reducing production of cholesterol in the liver. Garlic (*Allium sativum* L.) has a long history as a food with a unique flavor and aroma along with some medicinal qualities.

Scientific research has revealed that the wide variety of dietary and medicinal functions of garlic can be attributed to the organosulfur compounds present in or generated from garlic. Allicin is believed to be responsible for much of the antibacterial activity of garlic, while methyl allyl trisulfide is antithrombotic (preventing or interfering with the formation of blood clots), and diallyl trisulfide shows anticancer activity. Organosulfurs are also found in chives, leeks, onions, scallions and shallots.[11]

Saponins

Saponins are modified carbohydrates found in many vegetables and herbs that neutralize enzymes in the intestines that may cause cancer. Along with their anticancer activity, there is evidence that some saponins lower circulating levels of certain lipids. In the laboratory, saponins show a dose-response cytotoxic effect and an antiproliferative action on the cancer cells.[12] They also may help to strengthen the immune system and promote wound healing. Saponins are found in soybeans, whole grains, beans, and ginseng root, shown here. Researchers have identified eleven different saponins in soybeans alone.

Capsaicin

A component of certain plants, including cayenne and hot red pepper, capsaicin is used topically to relieve nerve pain. Capsaicin appears to act by reducing levels of substance P, a compound that contributes to inflammation and the delivery of pain impulses from the central nervous system. Research suggests that it has a profound antiproliferative effect on cancer cells, inducing apoptosis and inhibiting NF-kappa activation to slow the growth of cancer cells.[13]

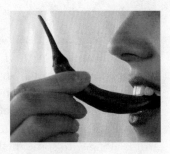

Sterols

Sterols, which include sitosterol, stigmasterol, campesterol, and squalene, are found in vegetable oils. Sitosterol is the most studied and appears to have cholesterol-lowering effects. Recent studies show that sterols (2 grams/day) lower LDL cholesterol and reduce biomarkers of oxidative stress and inflammation. Plant sterols probably exert their cholesterol-lowering effects by interfering with the uptake of both dietary and biliary cholesterol from the intestinal tract.[14]

Measuring Antioxidant Content and Activity

ORAC—oxygen radical absorbance capacity—is a key method of measuring the antioxidant capability of foods. ORAC is a standardized test developed by the National Institute on Aging and adopted by the U.S. Department of Agriculture to measure the total antioxidant potency of foods and nutritional supplements. The ORAC method has become the industry gold standard for measuring antioxidants. It is expressed as units per 100 grams of sample. Simply stated, the higher the ORAC value per equivalent weight of food, the more antioxidant power it contains.

Antioxidants Play a Key Role in Disease Prevention

Epidemiological studies, which consider the incidence and prevalence of disease in populations as opposed to individuals, have shown that low plasma levels of antioxidant micronutrients, which are commonly found in fruit and vegetables, are associated with increased risk for diseases such as heart disease, cancer and metabolic disorders. These studies also reveal that even health-conscious Americans often fail to obtain the recommended amount of fruit and vegetables in their diets.

One study tracked the dietary habits of a group of healthy middle-aged men and women to assess the effect of supplementation with a natural phytonutrient preparation from fruits and vegetables on plasma levels of various antioxidant micronutrients and oxidative stress. In a rigorous randomized double-blind study, researchers gave subjects a supplement or placebo for a total of 14 weeks. Blood levels of beta-carotene, vitamin C, vitamin E, selenium and folate were measured at 0, 7 and 14 weeks. Fruit and vegetable consumption was monitored using a food frequency questionnaire at weeks 0, 7 and 14. The research documented significant increases in blood nutrient levels after active supplementation with phytonutrients. Among the subjects who received the supplement, the ranges measured after supplementation often rose to those associated with a reduced risk for disease.[15]

Some researchers speculate that the chronic diseases that beset us as we age, such as diabetes, cancer, heart disease and Alzheimer's disease may be attributable to our lack of knowledge about the vital role of antioxidant phytonutrients in our diet. They assert that as we gain an understanding of phytonutrients and actively include adequate amounts of them in our diets, we may be able to prevent some of these chronic diseases in much the same way that diseases such as scurvy were eradicated by our appreciation of vitamin C requirements and deficiencies.

Antioxidants and Heart Health

Cardiovascular disease (CVD)—which includes coronary heart diseases, arrhythmias, diseases of the arteries, congestive heart failure, rheumatic heart disease, cerebrovascular disease (stroke), and congenital heart defects—is the leading cause of death in the United States. Heart disease is second only to all cancers combined in terms of deaths rate and years of potential life lost.

Since deficiencies in Vitamins A, C, E and beta carotene have been linked to heart disease, many researchers believe that taking antioxidants should benefit heart health. Further, antioxidant compounds found in fruit and vegetables, such as vitamin C, carotenoids and bioflavonoids, may influence the risk of CVD by preventing the oxidation of cholesterol in arteries. However, clinical research has produced conflicting results, and several studies have reported no reductions in heart disease among people who had taken antioxidant vitamins.

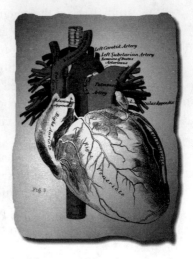

In 2003, the U.S. Preventive Service Task Force, an independent panel of experts in primary care and prevention that systematically reviews the evidence of effectiveness and develops recommendations for clinical preventive services, concluded that to date, the evidence is insufficient to recommend for or against the use of supplements of vitamins A, C, or E; multivitamins with folic acid; or antioxidant combinations for the prevention of cancer or cardiovascular disease.

But there is growing evidence of the effectiveness of specific bioflavonoids to reduce the risk of coronary heart disease. Italian researchers reported that a high intake of anthocyanidins reduced the risk of acute myocardial infarction (heart attack) even after allowances were made for consumption of alcohol, fruit and vegetables. Their research supported a real inverse association between consumption of this class of bioflavonoids and heart attack risk.[16]

Another study confirmed the heart-health benefits of the antioxidant effects of polyphenols in red wine. Patients with and without coronary artery disease were given red wine polyphenols for 14 days, and both groups experienced improvements in their coronary microcirculation. The investigators speculate that improved endothelial function (the endothelial cells line blood vessels, and their function determines blood vessel dilation) is the potential mechanism by which purple grape products may prevent cardiovascular events. The antioxidant effect of red wine polyphenols may improve coronary microcirculation by improving endothelial function.[17]

Recent epidemiologic studies have confirmed the relationship between antioxidants, particularly dietary and serum (blood levels) levels of carotenoids, and reduced cardiovascular disease and mortality. One study conducted in Japan concluded that high serum levels of total carotene, comprising alpha- and beta-carotenes and lycopene, may reduce the risk for cardiovascular disease mortality.[20]

Other research suggests that vitamin E is especially effective at reducing the inflammatory processes associated with the development of atherosclerotic plaque and ischemic heart disease. (IHD is characterized by weakened pumping action of the heart caused by a decreased blood supply from narrowing or occlusion of the coronary arteries.) [21]

Antioxidants and Stroke

Stroke (cerebrovascular disease) is a cardiovascular disease that affects the blood vessels of the central nervous system. When an artery supplying oxygen and nutrients to the brain bursts or becomes clogged with a blood clot, a part of the brain does not receive the oxygen it needs. Without the necessary oxygen, the affected nerve cells die within moments. The parts of the body controlled by these nerve cells also become dysfunctional. Because dead brain cells cannot be replaced, the damage done by a stroke is often permanent.

Stroke is the third leading cause of death in the Unites States, following heart disease and cancer. The Centers for Disease Control and Prevention (CDC) report that each year about five hundred thousand people suffer a new stroke and two hundred thousand have a recurrent stroke.

Oxidative stress has been implicated in the development of stroke as well as neurodegenerative diseases like Parkinson's and Alzheimer's disease, Huntington's disease and epileptic seizures. A healthy diet that features antioxidant-rich fruits and vegetables and is low in salt and saturated fats may significantly lower the risk for a first stroke, perhaps by helping to protect against high blood pressure and obesity—significant risk factors for stroke.

A Mediterranean diet, which is high in beneficial oils, whole grains, fruits, and vegetables and low in cholesterol and animal fat, has been shown to reduce stroke and myocardial infarction by 60 percent in four years compared with the American Heart Association diet. The effectiveness of the Mediterranean diet, when compared to other diets or to supplementation with selected antioxidants, may be attributable to the fact that it provides a wide range of antioxidant vitamins and phytonutrients from fruits and vegetables of all colors.[22]

Some research reveals protection from stroke from antioxidant vitamins and carotenoids, including beta carotene, lycopene and astaxanthin,[24] as well as melatonin, which, along with scavenging free radicals, also acts to regulate the activity and expression of antioxidant and pro-oxidant enzymes.[23]

There also is promising research about the cerebroprotective effects of resveratrol, the polyphenolic compound found in grapes, red wine, purple grape juice, peanuts and some berries. Animal studies suggest that high doses of resveratrol may decrease the risk of clot formation and atherosclerosis.[25, 26]

Antioxidants and Cancer

Cancer is a large group of diseases characterized by the uncontrolled growth and spread of abnormal cells. These cells may grow into masses of tissue called malignant tumors. The dangerous aspect of cancer is that cancer cells invade and destroy normal tissue.

The spread of cancer cells occurs either by local growth of the tumor or by some of the cells becoming detached and traveling through the blood and lymph systems to start additional tumors in other parts of the body. Metastasis (the spread of cancer cells) may be confined to a region of the body, but left untreated (and often despite treatment), the cancer cells can spread throughout the entire body, causing death. It is perhaps the rapid, invasive and destructive nature of cancer that makes it, arguably, the most feared of all diseases, although it is second to heart disease as the leading cause of death in the United States.

Oxidative stress is now recognized as an important causative factor in the development of several chronic diseases, including cancer, cardiovascular diseases, osteoporosis, and diabetes. Because many cancers are thought to be initiated by the effects of oxygen-free radicals on DNA, the antioxidant vitamins A, C and E and beta carotene have been extensively researched. To date, there is no evidence to support the use of individual supplements to protect against cancer, and there is evidence that high doses of some of these vitamins may even be hazardous.

Some studies have reported an association between low blood levels of antioxidant vitamins and a higher risk for cancer, however, with the exception of vitamin E protecting against the development of bladder cancer, supplementing the diet with antioxidant vitamins has not been shown to reduce risk. Other research findings report higher risks for melanoma and lung cancer with high antioxidant intake. Individual supplements, however, do not offer any advantage. There is evidence that beta-carotene supplements may increase the risk for lung cancer in smokers.

Numerous studies have reported that fruits and vegetables rich in carotenoids are associated with protection against many cancers. Epidemiological, tissue culture, and animal studies provide convincing evidence supporting the role of lycopene, found in tomatoes, in the prevention of chronic diseases including prostate, colon, lung and bladder cancer.[27]

Bioflavonoids have demonstrated several cancer preventive properties. In addition to antioxidant activity, these compounds may reduce abnormal cell growth and inflammation; help the body get rid of cancer-causing agents; and restore communication between different cells in the body. Bioflavonoids and polyphenols are coming under extensive study and analysis for their potential cancer-fighting properties. In one two-decade study, people who ate flavonoid-rich foods had a 20 percent lower risk for cancer in general. Resveratrol and quercetin have been found to have tumor-suppressing properties and some evidence suggests the genistein in soy may protect against lung cancer.

The organosulfur compounds found in the onion and garlic family may have very potent properties in suppressing or blocking carcinogenic substances. Epidemiological observations and laboratory studies, both in cell culture and animal models, have indicated the anticancer potential of garlic and its constituents, which has been traditionally used for varied human ailments throughout the world. Studies indicate that people who regularly consume fresh or cooked garlic have about half the risk of developing stomach cancer and two thirds the risk of colorectal cancer as people who eat little or no garlic. One possible explanation for garlic's anticancer effect in the stomach is its antibacterial action against *H. pylori*, which can promote stomach cancer.

There are several other mechanisms of action that may explain the cancer-preventive effects of garlic-derived products. These include modulation in activity of several metabolizing enzymes that activate and detoxify carcinogens and inhibit DNA adduct formation, antioxidative and free radicals scavenging properties and regulation of cell proliferation, apoptosis and immune responses. Recent data show that garlic-derived products modulate cell-signaling pathways in a manner that controls the unwanted proliferation of cells. These findings suggest that organosulfur compounds may have strong cancer preventive as well as cancer therapeutic effects.[30]

A tremendous amount of epidemiological research describing the potential role of antioxidant nutrients in the prevention of cancers has been amassed during the past few decades. However, results of large recent intervention trials do not support a preventive effect against cancer for supplementation with antioxidant nutrients.[29] The seemingly contradictory results reported by observational studies and clinical trials may be explained by the fact that the doses used in clinical trials were much higher than the highest levels attained by the usual dietary intake, which, in observational studies, were found to be associated with the lowest risk of cancer.

Another explanation of these research results may be that the effect of antioxidant supplementation on the incidence of cancer could depend on baseline (pre-treatment) antioxidant status, which varies based on gender and/or nutritional status and the overall health of subjects—healthy subjects as opposed to subjects considered at high risk for cancer. Antioxidant supplementation may have a beneficial effect on cancer risk and incidence only in healthy subjects who are not exposed to cancer risk and who have a particularly low baseline antioxidant status. High doses of antioxidant supplementation may be harmful in subjects in whom the initial phase of cancer development has already started, and they could be ineffective in well-nourished subjects with adequate antioxidant status.[28]

Antioxidants May Help to Slow Brain Aging

Several epidemiologic studies have found that vitamin E in food slows brain aging and protects against cognitive decline and the development of Alzheimer's disease (AD), which is a progressive, degenerative disease that affects the brain and results in severely impaired memory, thinking and behavior. It is the fourth leading cause of death in adults, and the incidence of the disease rises with age. AD is not a normal consequence of growing older, and researchers continue to seek its cause.

AD affects an estimated four million American adults and is the most common form of dementia, or loss of intellectual function. The U.S. Department of Health and Human Services estimates that 4.5 million Americans suffer from AD, and in 2004 it was the eighth-leading cause of death in the United States. AD also contributes to many more deaths that are attributed to other causes, such as heart and respiratory failure.

One ten-year study conducted at Vanderbilt University School of Medicine found that the risk of developing Alzheimer's disease was dramatically reduced for older people who drank fruit or vegetable juices regularly. The study reported that the incidence of Alzheimer's was 76 percent lower among subjects who drank juice three or more times a week compared to those who drank juice less than once a week. It was 16 percent lower for those drinking juice once or twice a week. The investigators attributed the findings specifically to polyphenols, rather than antioxidant content in general.[33]

Another recent study of healthy older adults found that consumption of leafy green vegetables, but not fruit consumption, was associated with a slower rate of cognitive decline as measured by assessment of recall, memory and other cognitive abilities. The study found that the slowdown in cognitive decline was greatest in the oldest people who ate at least two or more vegetable servings a day. Subjects who consumed two or more servings of vegetables a day had a 35 to 40 percent decrease in the decline in thinking ability over six years, which is comparable to being five years younger.[32]

Notes

1. Szeto YT, Chu WK, Benzie IF. Antioxidants in fruits and vegetables: a study of cellular availability and direct effects on human DNA. *Biosci Biotechnol Biochem.* 2006; 70(10): 2551–55.
2. Vinson JA et al. Polyphenols: total amounts in foods and beverages and U.S. per-capita consumption. Abstract number AGFD 10. Presented at the American Chemical Society 230th National Meeting in Washington, DC. August 28, 2005.
3. Baur JA et al. Resveratrol improves health and survival of mice on a high-calorie diet. Nature advance online publication 1 November 2006.
4. Omenn GS. Chemoprevention of lung cancer: The rise and demise of beta-carotene. *Annu Rev Public Health* 1998; 19: 73–99.
5. Bagchi D et al. Free radicals and grape seed proanthocyanidin extract: Importance in human health and disease prevention. *Toxicology.* 2000; 148: 187–97.
6. Shoskes DA, Zeitlin SI, Shahed A et al: Quercetin in men with category III chronic prostatitis: A preliminary prospective, double-blind, placebo-controlled trial. *Urology.* 1999; 54: 960–963.
7. Bhathena SJ, Velasquez MT. Beneficial role of dietary phytoestrogens in obesity and diabetes. *Am J Clin Nutr.* 2002 Dec; 76(6): 1191–201.
8. Tang L et al. Potent activation of mitochondria-mediated apoptosis and arrest in S and M phases of cancer cells by a broccoli sprout extract. *Mol Cancer Ther.* 2006; 5(4): 935–44.
9. Zhang Y, Yao S, Li J. Vegetable-derived isothiocyanates: anti-proliferative activity and mechanism of action. *Proc Nutr Soc.* 2006; 65(1): 68–75.
10. Grassmann J. Terpenoids as plant antioxidants. *Vitam Horm.* 2005; 72: 505–35.
11. Ariga T, Seki T. Antithrombotic and anticancer effects of garlic-derived sulfur compounds: a review. *Biofactors.* 2006; 26(2): 93–103.
12. Drissi A et al. Tocopherols and saponins derived from Argania spinosa exert, an antiproliferative effect on human prostate cancer. *Cancer Invest.* 2006; 24(6): 588–92.
13. Mori A et al. Capsaicin, a component of red peppers, inhibits the growth of androgen-independent, p53 mutant prostate cancer cells. *Cancer Res.* 2006; 66(6): 3222–9.
14. Devaraj S, Jialal I. The role of dietary supplementation with plant sterols and stanols in the prevention of cardiovascular disease. *Nutr Rev.* 2006 Jul; 64(7 Pt 1): 348–54.
15. Kiefer I et al. Supplementation with mixed fruit and vegetable juice

concentrates increased serum antioxidants and folate in healthy adults. *J Am Coll Nutr.* 2004; 23(3): 205–11.

16. Tavani A et al. Intake of specific flavonoids and risk of acute myocardial infarction in Italy. *Public Health Nutr.* 2006; 9(3): 369–74.

17. Hozumi T et al. Beneficial effect of short term intake of red wine polyphenols on coronary microcirculation in patients with coronary artery disease. *Heart.* 2006; 92(5): 681–82.

18. Taubert, D et al. Chocolate and Blood Pressure in Elderly Individuals With Isolated Systolic Hypertension. *J Am Med Assoc* 2003; 290(8): 1029–30.

19. Serafini, M et al. Plasma antioxidants from chocolate. *Nature.* 2003; 424: 1013.

20. Ito Y et al. Cardiovascular disease mortality and serum carotenoid levels: a Japanese population-based follow-up study. *J Epidemiol.* 2006; 16(4): 154–60.

21. Chattopadhyay A, Bandyopadhyay D. Vitamin E in the prevention of ischemic heart disease. *Pharmacol Rep.* 2006; 58(2): 179–87.

22. Spence JD. Nutrition and stroke prevention. *Stroke.* 2006; 37(9): 2430–35.

23. Suzen S. Recent developments of melatonin related antioxidant compounds. *Comb Chem High Throughput Screen.* 2006 Jul; 9(6): 409–19.

24. Hussein G et al. Astaxanthin, a carotenoid with potential in human health and nutrition. *J Nat Prod.* 2006 Mar; 69(3): 443–49.

25. Fukao H, Ijiri Y, Miura M, et al. Effect of trans-resveratrol on the thrombogenicity and atherogenicity in apolipoprotein E-deficient and low-density lipoprotein receptor-deficient mice. *Blood Coagul Fibrinolysis.* 2004; 15(6): 441–46.

26. Wang Z, Zou J, Huang Y, Cao K, Xu Y, Wu JM. Effect of resveratrol on platelet aggregation in vivo and in vitro. *Chin Med J.* 2002; 115(3): 378–80.

27. Rao AV, Ray MR, Rao LG. Lycopene. *Adv Food Nutr Res.* 2006; 51: 99–164.

28. Hercberg S, Czernichow S, Galan P. Antioxidant vitamins and minerals in prevention of cancers: lessons from the SU.VI.MAX study. *Br J Nutr.* 2006; 96 Suppl 1: S28–30.

29. Coulter ID et al. Antioxidants vitamin C and vitamin e for the prevention and treatment of cancer. *J Gen Intern Med.* 2006; 21(7): 735–44.

30. Shukla Y, Kalra N. Cancer chemoprevention with garlic and its constituents. *Cancer Lett.* June 20, 2006.

31. Vinson JA. Chocolate is a powerful ex vivo and in vivo antioxidant, an antiatherosclerotic agent in an animal model, and a significant contributor to antioxidants in the European and American Diets. *J Agric Food Chem.* 2006; 54(21): 8071–76.

32. Morris MC et al. Associations of vegetable and fruit consumption with age-related cognitive change. *Neurology.* 2006; 67: 1370-76.

33. Dai Q et al. Fruit and Vegetable Juices and Alzheimer's Disease: The Kame Project. *The American Journal of Medicine.* 2006; 119(9): 751–59.

34. Moeller SM et al. Associations Between Intermediate Age-Related Macular Degeneration and Lutein and Zeaxanthin in the Carotenoids in Age-Related Eye Disease Study (CAREDS): Ancillary Study of the Women's Health Initiative. *Arch Ophthalmol.* 2006; 124: 1151–62.

35. Combs GF, Clark LC, Turnbull BW. An analysis of cancer prevention by selenium. *BioFactors 14* 2001; 153–59.